AF811684

MENTAL ILLNESSES
AND
DISORDERS

Origin and liberation

– ALAIN TELLO ROBLEDO "Beingist" –

© **Alain Tello Robledo**
Author: Alain Tello Robledo - AtelTrainer
Editor: Alain Tello Robledo - AtelTrainer

First Edition: October 2022
Second Edition: September 2024

Interior layout: Chantal Tello García
Cover illustration and layout: Chantal Tello García
Proof-reading: Chantal Tello García
www.chantaltello.com

ISBN: 978-84-125819-3-5
Legal deposit (Spain): V-3301-2024

All rights reserved. Pursuant of falling into any of the sanctions set up in the applicable copyright laws, no part of this publication may be reproduced, stored or introduced into a retrieval system, or transmitted, in any form or by any means (electronic, mechanical, photocopying, recording or otherwise), without the prior written permission of both the copyright owner and the publisher of this book.

INDEX

Preface

Since Covid-19's forced confinements, emotional and mental disorders have skyrocketed around the world.

Every day, more people are admitted to psychiatric clinics, take anxiolytic treatments or fall into addictions (drugs - alcohol ...).

The fact that young people are the most affected is especially worrying, as they are the future of humanity. The loss of freedom forced by confinement has greatly shaken up the children of the world, who need to move freely in order to grow up.

As with any loss of freedom, it is easier for the most fragile side of Beings to emerge, thus causing suffering.

Social networks have become the escape valves into a virtual reality which hides economic interests, manipulation and expressions of humanitarian unrest.

More and more children are self-harming, substituting emotional pain for physical pain and drawing attention to their deep, existential despair. Suicide rates have also increased dramatically.

This book aims to help people to free themselves from any emotional or mental disorder, from the transformative understanding of transcendental "Beingist" knowledge.

Presentation

Alain Tello Robledo, founder of AtelTrainer, while being far from society, religions and beliefs for many years, has made it his life's mission to spread ancestral healing from transcendental knowledge, to free people and beings from suffering, illnesses and emotional and mental disorders.

As humanity recovers its well-being in union with Existence, the balance of ecosystems and life on Earth will undoubtedly be recovered.

Alain, born in 1961, suffered from chronic allergic asthma since a young age, from myopia since he was 30 years old, and from generalised anxiety with pharmacological treatment of "Trankimazin" (anxiolytics) for 16 years.
His deepest unrest made him leave society, friends and family around 2014-15, to isolate himself in the little Valley of Hortunas, Spain, where today exists the first

"Beingist" Center of Transcendental Knowledge and Ancestral Healing, which he built with his own two hands and the help of his wife Massiel and his daughter Chantal, who visit him on weekends to help him, as they trusted his intentions and intuition from the very beginning.

There, in the Valley of Hortunas, Spain, Alain developed the Essence to Essence Healing he calls Ancestral, and healed himself of all his illnesses and disorders, while also freeing and healing many other people who prepared themselves to receive the single ancestral treatment, some of which have shared their experiences of liberation on the website www.ateltrainer.com.

This publication answers Alain's need to share a knowledge that belongs to us all to help us be free, healthy, fearless, happy and at peace, through AtelTrainer.

Because humanity has moved away from transcendental common sense, we have created the world we have today, full of wars, diseases, climate and energetic change.

After hitting rock bottom, humanity is irrevocably going through the process of transcendental change, in order to regain its lost balance and health.

From my deepest feeling, in connection "with what cannot be seen", I can assure that the change towards the "New World - Coming very soon" (manuscript published at the end of 2021) will be materialised in a way which nothing and no one can stop the course of Existence towards life, evolution, creation and health.

Each person has the power to facilitate the transcendental change through small actions, but with an enormous universal consciousness, fuelled by the innate intentions of each of us which will be unveiled in each step towards understanding the unique reality of things.

The disbelief and resistance of inflexible people who have made this world ill, will not be able to stop the movements forced by Existence (climate changes, energy crises, pandemics), and the disappearance of the social system as we know it, to force humanity to change.

People will heal and free themselves from all their fears to live in harmony. They will be witnesses and protagonists of the future of new consciousness, wonderful for humanity, in union with all the Beings of the Planet.

Introduction

The objective of the present publication is to inform, from "Beingist" knowledge, about the causes of mental illnesses and disorders that, in our current times, are affecting more and more people, as well as explaining the mechanisms of liberation from transcendental knowledge and Ancestral Healing.

Mental disorders are defined as:
<<<< alterations in the processes of reasoning, behaviour, the ability to recognise reality, emotions or the relationship with others, considered abnormal with respect to the social reference group from which the person comes>>>>.

The evaluation of patients is done by psychiatry or psychology professionals. With their assessments and diagnoses based on analysis through observation of the patients' behaviour, actions and thoughts.
"Normal" is defined as everything that is accepted by the beliefs, values and actions of the reference groups (majority) studied through interpretations, according to the reality created by humanity itself.

Everything that is different from what is supposedly "normal" is considered "abnormal", thus labelling all "different" people as mentally ill.

Transcendental reflections

From the "Beingist" transcendental knowledge there are only two groups to define the normal and the abnormal:

- The "sane", that is, people who try to live in harmony with themselves and their environment, regardless of their beliefs, and whose actions are always backed by their intention and will to not bring harm to anyone, whether that be people, animals or environment, least of all themselves. They are sincere, noble, generous and fair.

- The "insane", i.e., people whose conscious and unconscious actions harm their environment, people, animals, ecosystems, and/or themselves.

The people belonging to the "insane" category are the only ones who should receive psychiatric and psychological help to prevent them from harming themselves or others.

The group of people nowadays considered as "not sane", as soon as they are diagnosed through dangerous actions which have either already taken place or are very likely to happen, are imprisoned through psychotic treatments in psychiatric centers, dehumanised in their majority.
In these cases, and also from the "Beingist" point of view, it is necessary to separate dangerous people, but in a provisional way, since there is the possibility of changes in the mental structure if they are "rehabilitated" in harmonious, humanised and creative environments.

However, some of these patients are victims of erroneous diagnoses and unjustly receive severe pharmacological incarceration for being sensitive and maladjusted to the current social reality which fosters injustice, violence and imbalance.
This social reality, whose political and economic system maintains inequalities among all beings is supported by beliefs opposed to the transcendental reality of the meaning of life. A social reality which this year 2022 shows us the final result of: wars between people, genocides, and destruction of ecosystems and the entire Planet.

Sensitive people who do not tolerate social nonsense, may be suffering from childhood nervousness, depression, generalised anxieties, etc., and even, at one point in their lives they may have attempted suicide, as a last resort to ask for help, motivated by despair, and for being people who could never harm others. These people receive the same diagnosis and treatment as people without empathy or with a mental dysfunction irreversible in the short-term.

A person who attempts suicide out of emotional desperation as a cry for help, cannot be diagnosed in the same way as a person who acts out of a mental disorder from a destructive, unsympathetic, violent and unconscious reality.
The causes of a suicide attempt by a chronically psychotic or depressed person are different, therefore their diagnoses and treatments must be different as well.

Addictions to drugs and alcohol, whether occasional or permanent, alienate the behaviour of addicted people, and the same happens to patients with severe mental dysfunction.
Humanity lives the opposite of the meaning of life. Life is not created to destroy or divide. Life is creation and union, since all beings in this world share the same destiny of the planet that sails at full speed through universal space.

No one is born to suffer or kill.

We are born to live in peace, freely and in harmony.

To share unselfishly is to help maintain the global balance, it is the perennial source of joy and satisfaction, it is transcendental love.

To live is to help the planet that helps us to be here, which is the basis of common sense and transcendental meaning of life. That is, to help the ecosystems, the flora and fauna. To live is to discover oneself in every circumstance.

Society is victimised for following the beliefs and inertia of a distant past that created a reality, the reality of humankind, which deviated from the meaning of life on this planet and birthed a society that has put in place a system of power and manipulation to benefit the "rich" minority and enslave the "poor and middle class"majority (mass).

The dark powers (minority) have established, using the people's fear of social exclusion, a system impossible to escape for the people who feed with their sweat, suffering and fear, the bank accounts of the "powerful" who do not hesitate to also ruin the planet to satisfy their need of power.

The "poor" dream of becoming rich in order to join the world's dominant side and escape the threat of social exclusion.

The dreams and ambitions of the majority of people are the reins of the powerful to control the masses, to continue enriching themselves without caring about how they are deeply damaging the planet and killing the future of the new generations to come. Selfishness is to blame for everything.

Society becomes an accomplice if it does not open its eyes and raise its consciousness to stop feeding the games of destructive power, to open the doors to the transcendental reality in union with all, favouring the arrival of the New World.

Since last century's industrial revolution, human knowledge has been rapidly evolving, but only materially, hand in hand with science, creating machines and mechanical processes that have contributed to making life easier for people.

Humankind's knowledge can repair the machines they manufacture, because they are their own creations, but they can never "fix" or "cure" the deep illnesses of the body and mind that were created by Existence herself, they can merely alleviate the symptoms. Only the Essences (Vital Energy) can do that. *Explained in detail in the fourth book, "Transcendental Love, Ancestral Healing"*.

Humankind's knowledge and beliefs have created a destructive lifestyle, misusing the genuine functioning of the body and mind, generating dysfunctions that have led to chronic and irreversible diseases by living disconnected from Vital Energies, just like a user breaks a machine for not having followed the manufacturer's guidelines for proper operation and maintenance.

Origin of diseases

The worst part is that the beliefs imposed by the powerful and assumed by the masses are embedded, generation after generation, in people's memory (DNA), because humanity deviated from its Existential path thousands of years ago, led by the hand of ancient civilisations which craved power, wealth and domination, such as:

- Ancient Egypt.
- Chinese Dynasty.
- Muslim expansion.
- Roman Empire.
- Ottoman Empire.
- Byzantine Empire.
- Aztec Empire.
- Inca Empire.
- Spanish Empire.
- British Empire.
- French Colonial Empire.
- etc.,

Ancient civilisations sowed the seed of desire for power, driven by absolute selfishness, whose fruits are bringing humanity and the entire planet to the brink of extinction.

In a more ancient past, prior to the birth of the aforementioned empires born of selfishness and antipathy, the natives lived in total self-sufficiency and respect for their environment. They lived in harmony with nature, with a true and sincere sense of generosity and hospitality. They were grateful for the land that fed them and the air they breathed, they venerated water as the most sacred thing, they sought to create their villages near springs. They only hunted out of necessity, to feed themselves, they did not kill for distraction, nor did they create thousands of excuses to ease their conscience, like modern hunters do. They lived in peace, united and happy. There was no such word as disease, there was only the word "wellbeing".

Today, most of the descendants of those natives of all continents who still survive are locked up in reservations or sleeping under unsanitary bridges, surviving on subsidies from the governing states as compensation or by begging. They soothe their suffering of "death in life" with alcohol and drugs, sometimes suicide being their only salvation from despair.

The genuine natives were generous, kind, happy.

It is said that when the first European settlers landed on the shores of New England (United States), they were welcomed with open arms by the Native Americans who had never seen the white man. The Natives' first reaction was one of surprise and welcome to the stranger.
But because of interests and the fight for "fur and gold", mainly occurring between France and England, the Indigenous Americans were manipulated into defending the interests of both sides, fighting each other for alcohol, guns and promises.

A few centuries later, as a result of the settlers' betrayal to the Natives, we can see which place Indigenous Americans and European settlers occupy in society today, both in the United States and Canada. The first dwellers are locked up in reservations, depressed, and the others who arrived later and were well received, ruling the lands of the First Americans.
The same happened in Australia, New Zealand, Africa, and other territories of the planet, not to mention the conquest of America by Spain, Portugal, England, France and the Netherlands.

Consequences

For centuries people have been conditioned, with obligations being the tribute to pay, in order to perhaps, one day, be able to achieve the dream instilled since childhood of being happy, the best, rich...?

Social exclusion, poverty, is the threat that keeps people in tension and perennial fear (anxiety), forcing them to do unwanted things (frustration), and even kill their neighbour (genocide - terror). These negative experiences and existential fears are a breeding ground for diseases, mental disorders and other pathologies.

Both anxiety and frustration have been added to people's daily lives for generations in the form of chronic stress.

This centuries-old generational fear, passed down from parent to child since ancient times, has weakened people's DNA.

Society as a whole is emotionally ill, to a greater or lesser extent, and in order to calm down some take or practice:

- ▷ Sleeping pills (addiction).
- ▷ Drugs (addiction).
- ▷ Alcohol (addiction).
- ▷ Tobacco (addiction).
- ▷ Pathological gambling (addiction).
- ▷ Video games (addiction).
- ▷ Social dependence (social networks - addiction).
- ▷ Work (excess-addiction).
- ▷ Sex (obsession-addiction).
- ▷ Sports (obsession-addiction).
- ▷ Eating (excess-obsession-addiction).
- ▷ Violence (consequence).

Children are forced to study hard in order to get a well-paying job. They are not given the opportunity to discover their vocation, to feel fulfilled as adults.

They are future adults with more or less professional success, but they will feel empty and frustrated at some point in their lives, when they are no longer so competitive, or when personal, material or family problems arise. No matter what achievements and possessions they have acquired, they will never free their silenced consciences.

But minds, in order to protect themselves from negative situations or emotions, can develop an antipathetic, narcissistic, selfish profile, addicted to all kinds of drugs, in order to have no remorse in climbing, at whatever cost, the rungs of success, exhausting themselves more and more over the years due to the enormous and unbalanced effort necessary to achieve their goals.

Other people will develop anxiety or depression because they are more sensitive and greatly empathetic, reinforced by their own Essences, because their lives are anchored to an unjust and inhuman system and their hearts are connected to the harmony and peace of nature, Existence.
Their emotional problems are the voices of their Essences asking for a change in their lives, because this world needs to listen to their silenced voices.

Others, as soon as they open their eyes at birth, become silent towards their social environment and their family (autism...) for having been born in a senseless world, not in a world as it should be. They only smile in contact with the purity and nobility of animals and nature. Their hearts will open when the New World appears, soon.

Others, like caged boars, have minds that can't stop and stand still, unable to concentrate because they are in an unbalanced, mindless environment (ADHD - impulsive behaviours - problems to focus - excess activity).

Others, as they are very mental people, unconsciously fall into narcissism. Personal, professional and social successes sharpen their chronic egotistic beliefs and behaviours.

Others, because of so much stress accumulated in their DNA since past generations, suffer ruptures in their neuronal chains, resulting in severe disorders such as schizophrenia, bipolarity, etc. and thus suffering more from social stigma. But it is important to know that there is a type of schizophrenia that is not originated by a mental failure, but by a gift to communicate with other dimensions. These people were and are the guides, healers, in ancient and modern primitive tribes.

Others, also because of the amount of stress accumulated in their DNA, and because they were born in a globalised environment of endless dangers and unconscious negative memories full of existential fears, manifest temporary or chronic paranoid episodes.

Observation and understanding

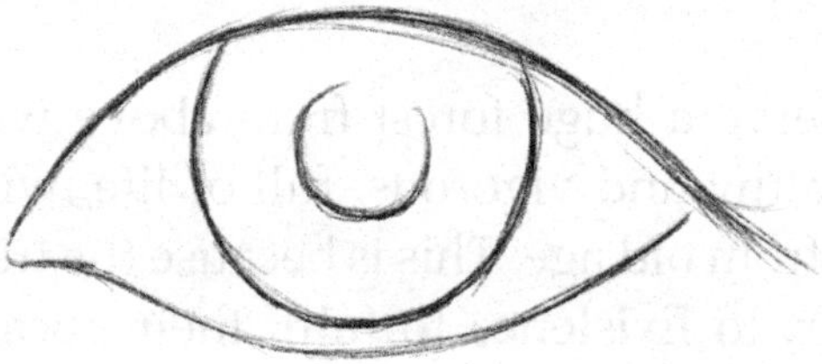

More important than being cured or healed, is to live in a balanced way so that our organism, body, mind and organs function optimally (prevention).

The modern human thinks and exhaust their body according to their mental wills and whims, based on personal interests or beliefs or advice from third parties, because they have lost the sensitivity to listen to the functional needs of their body-organism, Heart-Essence.

Living from the feeling and spontaneity of innate good intentions, is the best plan for maintaining health, and the best universal vaccine against all evils, as it does not block the passage of Vital Energy through the seventh chakra (*explained in detail in the fourth book "Transcendental Love, Ancestral Healing"*).

Among all diseases, there is only one that we cannot heal, it is the disease of the final departure. The other illnesses from a young age are illnesses of inherited and adaptive origin due to living against the feeling of our own Existence in our bodies and minds (emotions), and for living under the mantle of fear caused by worldwide violent economic and social systems.

If we observe a huge forest from above we will see it green, healthy and vigorous, full of life, with very few trees sick from old age. This is because the trees abandon themselves to Existence to fulfil their vocational function of tree, with their roots stuck deep in the earth (feet), their branches stretched out towards the sky (arms) and their crown looking at the stars (head).
Trees look the same from a distance, but each tree has its own function to keep the unity of the forest alive and healthy, contributing to maintain the existing balance of the Planet (oxygen, food, protection, etc.).
If humanity were a forest, from above we would see it gray, dark, sick, as people suffer from all kinds of problems hidden behind appearances. Some suffer from chronic illnesses, others from bone and joint problems, others from mental illnesses, and the majority, to a greater or lesser extent, are victims of worries, fears and anxieties that force them to silence their emotional discomforts in search of ephemeral peace.
People are lost because they have been distanced from their native identities, and from being able to materialise

their life missions. Each person is here as a puzzle piece to make a humanity united among itself, and among all the beings of the Planet, in order to guarantee the global existential balance and joy for future generations.

To a greater or lesser extent, all of humanity is mentally and emotionally ill from maintaining lifestyles that harm and kill their environment.

Is it "normal", is it intelligent, that human beings destroy each other (genocide), and destroy the ecosystems which keep them alive?

If the human reality and their beliefs were the only true ones, it would not destroy the future of new generations!

Who is crazier, the depressed, the sad, the anxious, the autistic person, or the "normal" people who fight to the death to maintain their destructive and separatist lifestyle? Not to mention the people who support wars and genocides for geopolitical interests.

Humanity has only evolved from a material standpoint, to make people's lives easier, enjoying more free time. But people have taken over free time and transformed it to continue feeding passive attitudes, distracted, destructive, not creative at all. Distractions and lifestyles that trample on Nature in all her magnitude, moving people away from their Essence and life missions.

The transcendental evolution is governed by the only changing reality of the Universe, of things, and of the Planet, alleviating the burdens of the ancestors' hard work with properly employed modern technology, to be able to enjoy more free time and live in union with the planet and all her beings, letting themselves be guided by life to live happy, free and in peace, for an indefinite period of time.

Existence gives us an increasing life expectancy, but we waste it in suffering, wars, diseases and fear of ageing, by living from a destructive reality.

Because humanity has evolved, generation after generation, only from its mental, rational and selfish side, following the erroneous beliefs of ancient civilisations that have created divided, unjust, and violent societies with a very superficial sense of happiness, new generations replicate the mistakes of the past, due to the memories embedded in their DNA.

Today's children are born into an unbalanced and superficial world, a polluted and sick Planet, which amplifies the fears inherited from the past and whose social stress has weakened people's neuronal and immunological systems, opening the door to diseases and mental disorders, not to mention adaptive diseases, such as çancer, allergies, etc.

With so many inherited traumas, people have been domesticated for centuries, submitted to existential fear. They have been losing the self-esteem and vital force necessary to recover the balance and freedom of all, showing clear vulnerability, falling prey to diseases and mental disorders.

People are caged behind the bars of systems filled with rules, laws, obligations, beliefs, castes, and inculcated fears.
Democracies are merely larger cages than dictatorships. We already know what happens to an animal locked up against their will in a cage, they become sick and go crazy because they have lost their freedom and connection with the outside world, their ability to live freely, to express themselves.

There are people who are aware of their mental and emotional disorder and ask for help.

There are people who do not know that they are conditioned at a subconscious level to not let their consciousness emerge, impeding their fears and emotional, sometimes mental, disorders from manifesting, whose actions favor the planetary imbalance. These people are the majority.

Since 2008, political and economic systems have been collapsing. Already in 2022 we can perceive the beginning of the decline of the humanity's world order as we know it, and the destruction of the Planet (ecosystems) due to human selfishness and ignorance, without any precedent in past times. A result of the evolution of minds to the detriment of Existential evolution.

Children are born without a future. Adults struggle to survive in our broken societies. Mental illnesses and disorders are more easily activated in hostile environments. Chronic despair invites suicide. Existential frustrations are relieved by a thousand distractions and addictions.

Having lived through so many centuries of repression, injustice, violence, fears and betrayals through past generations, the memories and neural links of human minds have been damaged.

Human minds by nature are conservative, distrustful and fearful, for having been witnesses of oppression, threats and insecurity for centuries; but if they had lived so many centuries in a free, generous and harmonious world the minds would be free, generous, harmonious, happy and balanced.

The only culprit of all evils is the many centuries of unconsciousness.

People are not directly guilty of the destruction of the planet, they are victims of so many centuries of oppression and globalised disunity.

However, people who do harm cannot be accepted or tolerated. Their indefinite separation from the masses is inevitable in order to give them a chance to free themselves, from the opening of their consciousness.

As all of humanity is once again immersed in a globalised environment of freedom, respect, union, existential security, health and peace, the new generations will live free, happy, healthy, in peace, and in harmony with the All.

Let's change now!

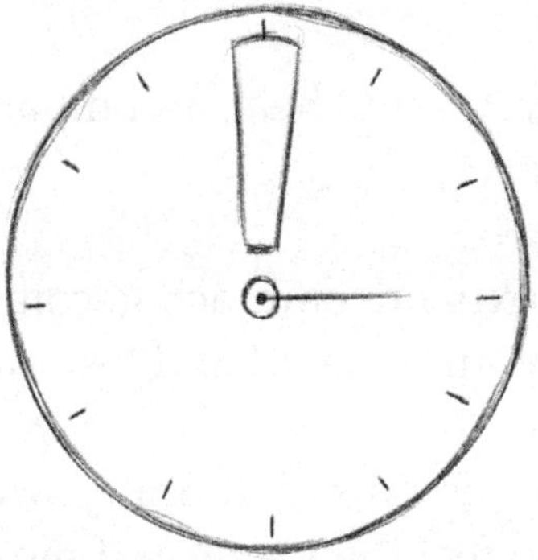

The change will either be voluntary or forced by the hand of Existence.

Understanding the flaws of the current values and beliefs is the only factor necessary to propel the elevation of consciousness, from the deep feeling, and realise that we have turned the paradise of the Universe into an inferno.

Connect with the transcendental knowledge that will open you to the universal reality of union between all Beings of the Planet, without interpretations.

Your enemy will become your friend and accomplice when you look together hand in hand at the horizon of the same destiny that unites all beings of the planet.
The quarrels of the past will only be long-forgotten memories, hidden in a remote corner of the mind, which will fade away with the focus on the New World of union that is coming.

Your mind will relax and heal, accompanied by a sincere and solemn smile.

Your heart will expand, embracing, comforting, guiding and protecting your agitated and lost mind.

Your mind-body-Essence will unite, sweeping away all fears, to begin to feel the magic and meaning of life and the Universe.

Your health will improve, knowing that there is a very simple and easy way to reach reality, obliterating all fear of an uncertain future.
It is time for hope and illusion to become reality. There is no turning back.

There is home, food, water and air available for all beings on the Planet, so they can live healthy, united, free, relaxed and happy.

There is excitement to travel to and enjoy every corner of the Planet, the home of all, harmoniously and without borders.
Existence is already taking the reins to make it so.

We are already seeing the changes on a planetary level, preparing people for a new consciousness, for the New World that is coming.

Free manuscript of The New World written from the Essences available at www.ateltrainer.com.

AtelTrainer's mission is to spread the transcendental and universal knowledge that belongs to all of us, far from religions and beliefs.

AtelTrainer's mission is to transmit Ancestral Healing in union with scientific medicine.

The inspiration of "Weare" - Alain Tello Robledo - and the AtelTrainer team is the transcendental and universal union between all Beings with the Planet (humans, fauna, flora...). Union that we call "Beingism".

Liberation & Healing

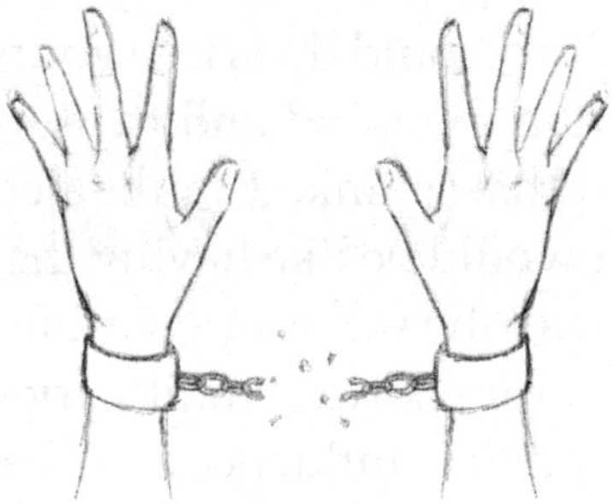

As I have commented and explained before, people are victims of the past of so many ancient civilisations, thus inheriting centuries of "existential stress".

Every person, without exception, manifests at any age disorders, limitations or diseases, which prevent them from living fully and making this wonderful world flourish again.

To quell the symptoms of imbalances, some go to doctors and take medication, others relax by drinking or eating excessively, a few more by smoking, some by practicing intense sports based on ibuprofen, a few by locking themselves indoors, and others by taking drugs.

As we can see, society as a whole is affected by imbalances, whose severity will manifest at different ages depending on: inherited genetic factors, family, social and professional environment, beliefs, healthy or unhealthy habits, obsessions and addictions, and the inner strength of each person.

The first thing you should do is free yourself from all beliefs, to reprogram the mind and the functioning of the nervous system that is linked to the needs and mental conditioning. It would be like having the intention to lovingly throw away the pages of your life journal written so far by others (memories, family, friends, education, norms, values, advice, influences...), to rewrite it yourself, from your own deepest feeling and with the intention to discover and follow your life's mission, your identity, your Essence, to open the passage of the Vital Energy through your seventh chakra, as explained in the fourth book "Transcendental Love Ancestral Healing".

It is necessary to swap rational knowledge, which is full of so much knowledge and beliefs that have divided societies and have led us to so much suffering, for transcendental, universal and liberating knowledge, which belongs to all of us.
First, one must have the firm intention to change, to honestly be oneself, free, independent and united with the Existence. The deep intention of sincere union with the

Planet and all her Beings, is what will guide you towards your liberation and Existential meaning.

For example, wishing to be healthy in order to be happy is not an intention, it is a desire of the selfish mind.

The transcendental intention is to give more priority to the universal unity, to your life's mission, rather than to yourself.

Put another way:

- ▷ If you make things good for the balance and union of the Planet and all the Beings that inhabit it, the Planet and Existence will take care of you. For this, the mind has to learn to abandon its desires and selfish programming, connecting with the faith in oneself (Essence), away from religions and beliefs.

- ▷ But if what you do is only for your own well-being, even if you wish to be generous afterwards to calm down your conscience, it is not the same. The mind wants to control and this action will close the access of the Vital Energy through the seventh chakra, as explained in AtelTrainer's book IV.
  To live is to let oneself be surprised by Existence, not to try to control it, because it is

infinite and manifests in a dimension impossible to understand from rational minds.

Preparation to free yourself from countless centuries of negative programming:

First of all, let the universal transcendental knowledge penetrate, move and relocate in the deepest part of your mind, and then your subconscious will relax, eliminating the inherited and inculcated negative neuronal programming gently and gradually.
A deep and lasting relaxation (peace of mind) can only happen when the mind's will is coherent with the Essence's mission.

Steps to follow:

1. Visit, from the heart, the website www.ateltrainer.com and pay attention to what deep feeling it brings you. You have to know that both AtelTrainer and Universal Transcendental Knowledge never tell or condition people to do things; they only help people to feel their life's intentions, to be themselves. In fact, you can only visit the AtelTrainer Beingist Center once for the sole ancestral healing treatment, if necessary.

2. Read the AtelTrainer website quietly from the heart to feel.

3. Take the free 44-minute pre-treatment, listening to the author's notes on "Good and Evil" while lying down peacefully.

4. Read all of the free author's notes (*https://www.ateltrainer.com/en/authors-notes/*).

5. Listen to all of the free audio author's notes (*https://www.ateltrainer.com/en/authors-notes/ or in the YouTube channel - Playlist of Alain Tello Robledo*).

6. Read the free manuscript on the New World (*web https://www.ateltrainer.com/en/the-new-world/*).

7. Practice daily and for a few minutes (3 to 7) the Transcendental Beingist Healing Meditation explained at *https://www.ateltrainer.com/en/transcendental-healing-meditation/*

8. Read the books on transcendental knowledge in chronological order (1, 2, 3, 4, 5, 6), all of them available on Amazon by searching for "Alain Tello Robledo". The purchase of the books will reinforce your change from thinking to feeling, but it will also help us to be able to continue our outreach on a planetary level, through the AtelTrainer Foundation (Transcendental Clinics and Hospitals of Ancestral Healing).

Many people have been deeply liberated so far, and their lives have changed after following the Ancestral Healing preparation for several months, feeling an opening of their heart and deep mental relaxation.

Program to prepare you to free yourself from addictions at *https://www.ateltrainer.com/en/do-you-want-to-free-yourself-from-your-addiction/*

♥♥♥

I am sure that after reading this publication and truly following the recommendations for the preparation of the Ancestral Healing treatment you will feel much better, and this improvement will become even greater as you connect with the feeling in your daily practice.

The recommended readings and audios will most probably make you feel good, but don't worry if you find yourself sometimes moved or troubled, no matter how little or how much that is, since while liberation is occurring strange sensations can sometimes be felt. If it happens just lie down, put your hands on your chest and belly button, relax your body, and abandon yourself in a long deep sigh from the intention of "I am not afraid, I trust my Essence", and it will soon pass.

AtelTrainer Ancestral Healing is complementary to Scientific Medicine, not an alternative.

Thank you!
Transcendental love hug to you!

"Weare" - Alain Tello Robledo - Beingist
& the AtelTrainer's Team

Other books from the author

Book I — Psycho-Fitness Holistic

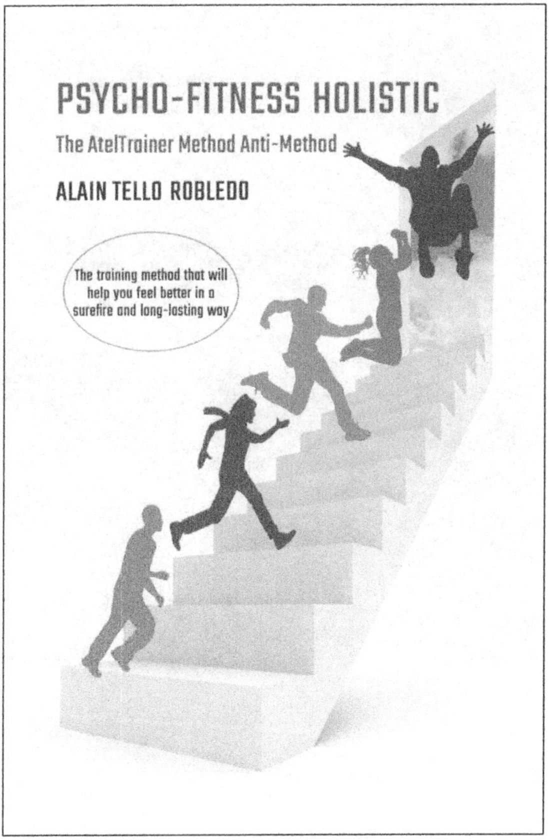

Book II — Zen Sport

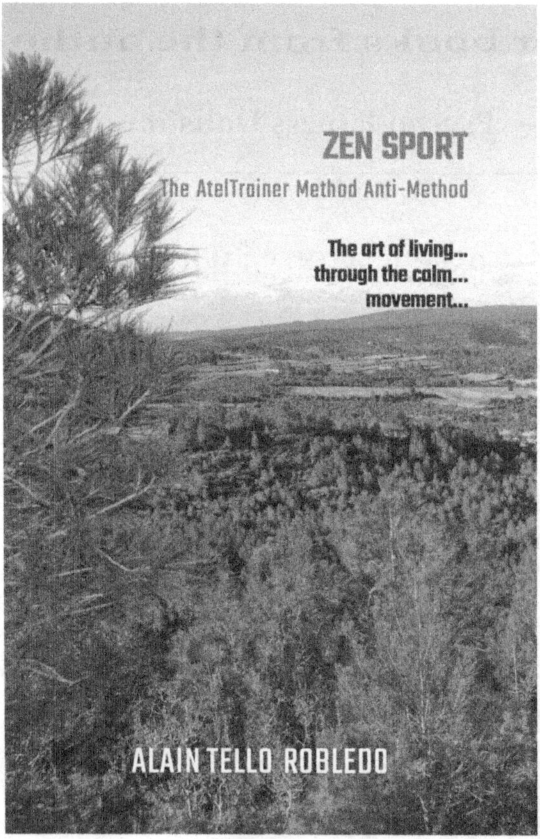

Book III — Transcendental Training

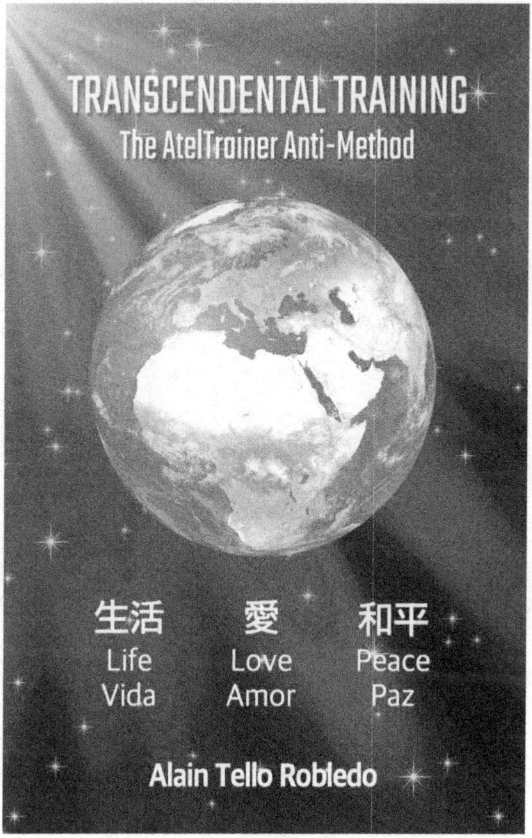

Book IV — Transcendental Love – Ancestral healing

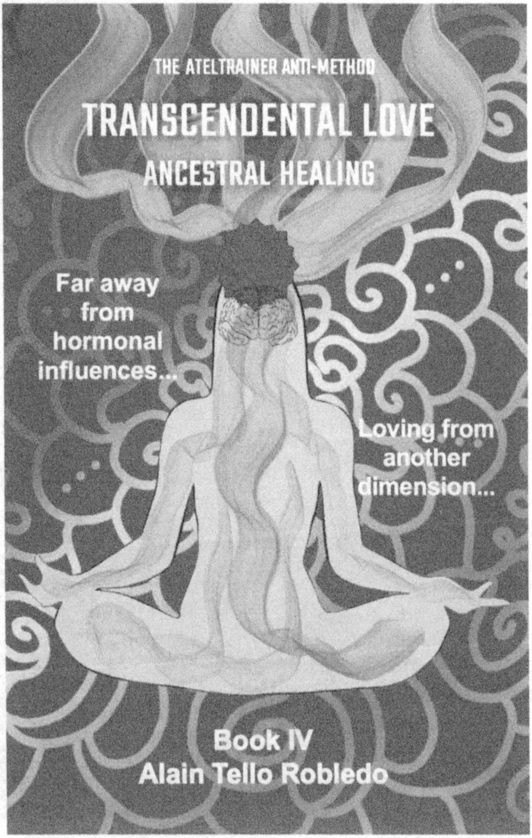

Book V — New World, Coming very soon !

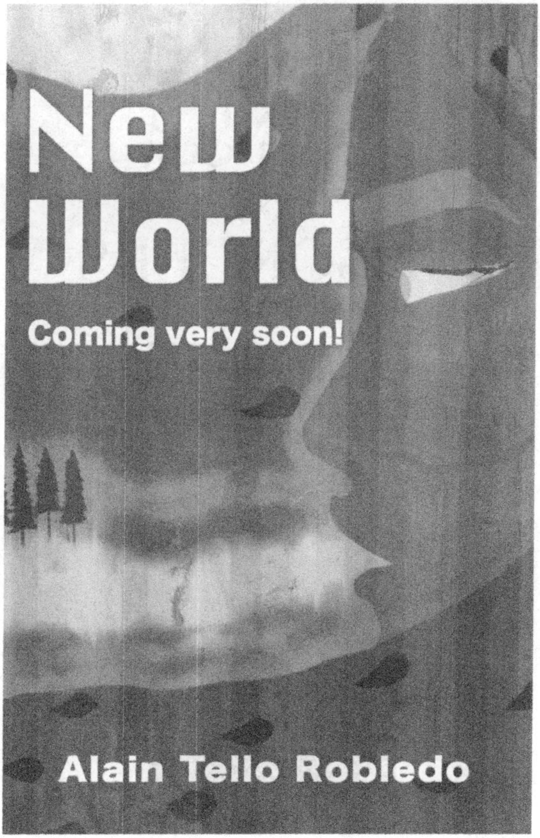

Book VI - The Origin of Mental Illnesses…

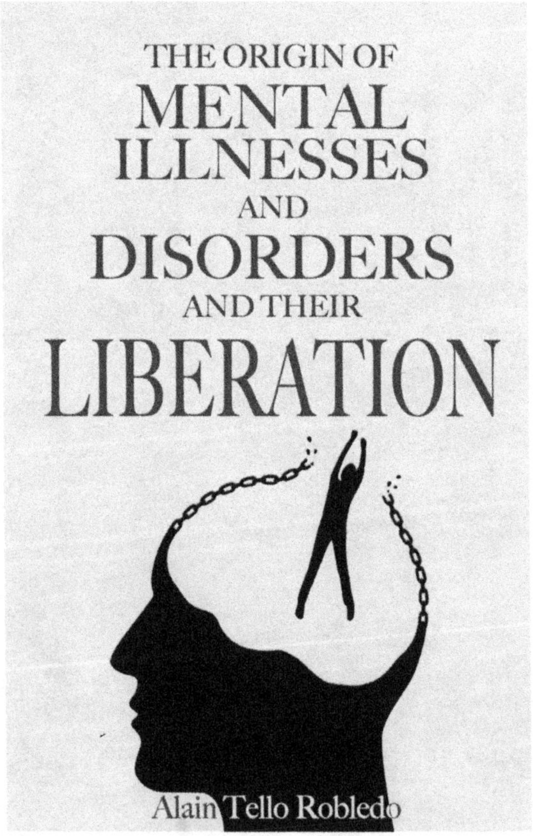

Book VII - The Stories of Bernard

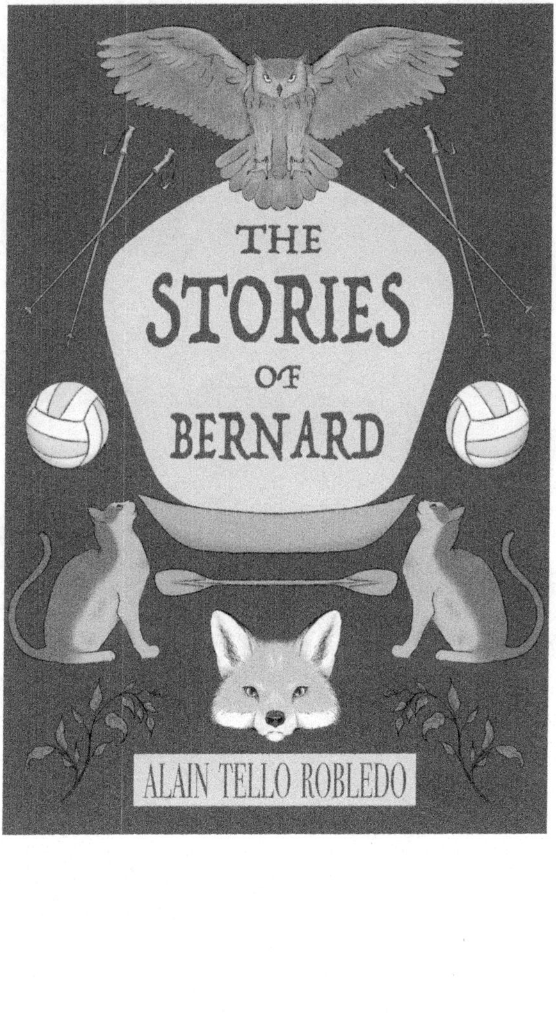

Made in the USA
Monee, IL
04 November 2026

67386413R10036